9 WAYS TO IMPROVE YOUR GUT HEALTH.

AUTHOR: DAVID RICHARD

Terms and Conditions

this publication, the Publisher assumes no responsibility for errors, omissions, or contrary interpretations of the subject matter herein. Any perceived slights of specific persons, peoples, or organizations are unintentional.

In practical advice books, like anything else in life, there are no guarantees of income made. Readers are cautioned to reply on thein their judgment about their circumstances to act accordingly.

Table of Contents

INTRODUCTION

There are tons of amazing importance of keeping your gut healthy, which you might have come across before reading this book. A healthy gut can make your digestion smooth, keep you away from a host of bad diseases, and also away from your doctor.

Our stomach contains a large **MICROBIOME** filled with bacteria that aids in properly digesting the food we eat. Some food and habits help to maintain healthy gut **MICROBIOMES,** while others can completely destroy your gut health. In this book, we will discuss habits and practices that will naturally help you to improve your gut health, which will make you live a healthy life.

ANTIBIOTIC ABUSE

Antibiotic abuse can prevent a healthy gut.

Antibiotics are life-saving medications that have a significant place in our world today, due to things we are exposed to. They frequently treat several ailments from sore throats to life-threatening illnesses in our bodies. **ANTIBIOTICS** works by creating antibodies that destroy both the harmful and helpful **MICROBIOTA** in the body or inhibit their reproduction and spread across the body. Regardless of how useful **ANTIBIOTICS** is, just a single course of treatment can result in the gut microbiota being infected by it. Sometimes, antibiotics use can increase the number of harmful bacteria like **CLOSTRIDIUM** and reduce the good bacteria like **LACTOBACILLI.** Gut flora is constantly affected by antibiotics. Even though the number of bacteria bounces back within a few weeks of treatment, they do not reach back to normal levels within the gut. Sometimes, the effect of antibiotics use can last up to two years even if the use was only short-term. So, after every use, we must take every necessary step to ensure that our gut flora return to normal. It is best to avoid unnecessary antibiotic consumption for every condition and only take it when the doctor prescribed it for you.

REDUCE STRESS

Our way of life, job, family, relationship, and society can tend to have a large impact on stress in our life which can distort our health. Excess stress is a major killer of gut microbiota. A stressed body can lead to a decreased blood flow into the gut, which can kill most of the bacteria in the gut and invariably alter the gut microbiota for the worse. Studies on mice show that increased stress can lead to a proportionate decrease in good gut bacteria and an increase in bad bacteria such as **CLOSTRIDIUM.** Studies on humans have shown a substantial decrease in the level of good bacteria like **LACTOBACILLI** with excessive stress levels, so reduced stress can contribute to an increase in the good gut bacteria.

To experience this, I will advise you to try stress-relieving exercise or yoga to relieve you of stress which will give you the best result you can ever imagine. Several studies emphasize the importance of good **gut flora.**

If your job is always stressful and there is no way to reduce it, I will advise you to always go for a medical check-up.

DIET

Having diversity in your diet can be healthy for your gut, but doing the opposite can be dangerous to your gut.

A balanced and diverse diet is necessary if we need to improve our gut health. Not having a wide range of foods and limiting one's diet to only processed sugar-rich food can significantly damage your gut flora and cause obesity which can affect your health. Dietary diversity is needed to maintain a proper gut **MICROBIOME**. Typically, fiber-rich whole grains, legumes, and some healthy food like yogurt have a long way to go in improving the gut health of its consumers, but the present diet of most people consists of minimal plant and animal proteins. A statistic reveals that a whopping 75 percent of AMERICAN's diet comes from a few sources of protein and vegetables. The deprivation in the diet can lead to horrible consequences for the gut bacteria, and the only way to remedy these issues is by eating more wholesome foods and keeping away from processed as much as possible.

PROBIOTICS

The easiest and most efficient way to improve your gut health is by incorporating **PROBIOTICS** into your diet. Probiotic food contains added bacteria that are beneficial for your gut health. It helps with metabolism but does not colonize your gut but needs to be consumed regularly for the best result. Probiotic food must not be negotiable. They promote the growth of healthy gut bacteria because they are food that breaks down through the bacteria in the gut. Probiotics are beneficial for the prevention of certain disorders such as heart disease and **TYPE 2 DIABETES**. Probiotic foods are incredibly beneficial for maintaining and healthy gut and preventing disease which will improve your overall health. Some probiotic foods are onion, garlic, asparagus, oats, cocoa, and flaxseed which are rich in polyphenols to keep your gut clean and robust. Polyphenols are plant-based **MICRONUTRIENTS** digested by our gut bacteria. Polyphenols provide a lot of health benefits, including a reduction in blood pressure, cholesterol levels, obesity, and inflammation, along with which they reduce excess stress.

For instance, dark chocolate, a food rich in polyphenols, has been shown to reduce the levels of inflammation in the human body. Red wine is also rich in polyphenols. In moderation, red wine can do wonders for the human gut, significantly in terms of improving the number of beneficial bacteria. I will also employ you to eat onions, cocoa, grape skins, green teas, and blueberries to improve your gut **MICROBIOTA**.

 Adding them to your daily diet through food like yogurt, or probiotic supplement after consulting your physio is good for your health.

ALCOHOL

Heavy alcohol intake needs to be watched because it can lead to addiction and eventually unexpected illness. Alcohol consumption especially heavy consumption can be harmful to your gut.

Alcohol is an intoxicant, which when consumed excessively can lead to a person losing their overall sense of time and place, sometimes even passing out.

Consumption of alcohol in excess is harmful to our bodies, and it can affect our liver and gut health by causing **INFLAMMATION.** Alcohol abuse can cause unexpected diseases as earlier said such as stroke, heart attacks, and even dementia over a long period.

However, alcohol in moderation and the consumption of certain types of alcohol like red wine can surprisingly promote the growth of healthy gut bacteria and prevent the development of harmful gut bacteria such as **CLOSTRIDIUM.** The benefits of red wine on gut health are from the presence of **POLYPHENOLS** in it.

POLYPHENOLS are beneficial to your gut health as they do not break down during digestion but are broken down by gut bacteria, making them valuable for their proliferation.

Alcohol stands in the grey area as excessive intake is bad for your overall health, but some types of alcohol in moderation can be very beneficial for your gut health.

Alcohol can be a tool for enjoyment and excitement among your friends if taken moderately, but can also damage your gut health terribly if taken excessively.

SMOKING

Some habits and certain lifestyle choices can be detrimental to your overall digestive health, and certain habits can create a lot of bacteria in your gut such as smoking. **Smoking** is a dreadful killer habit for your gut health. It can cause several disorders ranging from heart attacks, strokes, lung disease, and sometimes cancer. **Smoking** is especially bad for your gut **MICROBIOMS** as it destroys **gut flora**. It can also cause several gut disorders, such as **INFLAMMATORY BOWEL** disease, a severe condition where the intestines are inflamed hindering digestion.

The best way to improve gut flora and restore your health is to quit smoking immediately because it is harmful to your health. If you can't stop smoking immediately, have a long-term plan on how you will stop which am sure will work for you.

FERMENTED FOOD

Fermented food makes your gut strong. They are another premium source of healthy gut bacteria. Fermented food is mostly complex sugars that break down into simpler sugars, yeast, or bacteria. Most fermented food is rich in **LACTOBACILLI** which is beneficial for overall gut health. Studies by Pub.Med.gov, show that fermented food like yogurt increases the level of good bacteria such as **LATOBACILLI** in the system while reducing the level of micro-organisms that cause inflammation.

Yogurt also reduces symptoms of lactose intolerance in consumers. It's best if yogurt consumers refrain from having flavored yogurt as they usually contain very unhealthy levels of added sugar. It's always best to stick to the plain and unsweetened variety of yogurt. Choosing enhanced fermented foods with bacterial calories will help consumers make the most out of their fermented food which I will personally advise you to add to your diet. Some popular fermented foods are Kefir, Kombucha, and Tempeh.

EATING WHOLE GRAIN

Whole grain is a rich source of fiber, and fiber is essential for the microbiomes in your gut. Apart from fibers, whole grains also contain indigestible carbs broken down by bacteria. Studies by Pub.Med.gov, show that consuming whole grains can increase the number of good bacteria like **LACTOBACILLI** in your gut. They also show that consuming whole grains which are rich in beta-glucan (a non-digestible carbohydrate) can improve the levels of safety, as well as reduce the risk of cardiovascular diseases by altering the gut microbiota. Whole grains are not suitable for everyone, especially those who are gluten intolerant. It is advisable to check with your doctor or dietician before incorporating gluten-rich food into your diet.

EAT FRUITS AND VEGETABLES

Fruits, vegetables, and legumes are fiber-rich foods. Consuming fiber-rich foods leads to an increase in the number of beneficial gut bacteria. Studies show that a diet rich in fruit can prevent the growth of disease-causing bacteria in the human body.

Studies also show that at least fruits like almonds, apples, and **PISTACHIOS** have increased the level of helpful bacteria that prevent inflammation. Fruits and vegetables that are good for maintaining a healthy gut flora include bananas, apples, green peas, broccoli, raspberries, artichokes, and lentils.

Do not hesitate to start eating foods, fruits, and vegetables that are suitable for you, and try staying clear of habits that are not good for your health like drinking and smoking excessively. Are you going to adopt any of these ways to make your gut healthy? I will be tremendously excited if you do so. **HEALTHY HEALTH, HEALTHY LIFE.**

9 798393 051143